Before All Dignity Is Lost

The Living and Dying of an AIDS Victim

NORMAN R. BEAUPRÉ

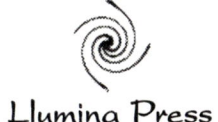

Llumina Press

© 2006 Norman R. Beaupré

All rights reserved. No part of this publication may be reproduced or transmitted in any form or by any means electronic or mechanical, including photocopy, recording, or any information storage and retrieval system, without permission in writing from both the copyright owner and the publisher.

Requests for permission to make copies of any part of this work should be mailed to Permissions Department, Llumina Press, PO Box 772246, Coral Springs, FL 33077-2246

ISBN: 1-59526-620-8

Printed in the United States of America by Llumina Press

Library of Congress Control Number: 2006907801

By the Same Author

L'Enclume et le couteau-----the Life and Work of Adelard Coté folk artist, NMDC, Manchester, N.H., 1982.

Le Petit Mangeur de Fleurs, Chicoutimi, Éd. JCL, 1999.

Lumineau, Chicoutimi, Éd. JCL, 2002.

Marginal Enemies, Llumina Press, Coral Springs, FL, 2004

Deux Femmes, Deux Rêves, Llumina Press, Coral Springs, FL, 2005.

La Souillonne, monologue sur scène, Llumina Press, Coral Springs, FL, 2006.

My dignity is borne off on the wind,
and my welfare vanishes like a cloud.

> Job 30:16-17

With deep affection for,
and in memory of,
the real "Drew"

Prologue

A I D S kills. Fills with terror the very soul of existence. It crushes hopes, annihilates dreams and devastates the lives of those left behind. But, one thing it doesn't do, it does not diminish the courage of living and dying. There are some remarkable cases where the human spirit soars above illness and pain, depression and the letting go, as well as the treacherous indignity attached to an infection for which there is yet no cure. However, AIDS stirs to compassion those who witness and those who pray. AIDS also bolsters the resolve of those of us who will not give up the struggle to spread compassion and rekindle the fire that burns bright with hope. With steadfast determination to do one's share in the healing process, those who wait and truly care become part of the healing. Healing is both for those afflicted with AIDS and those who share the anguish and suffering of its victims. I know. I have found some measure of healing in my relationship with Drew who went through the harrowing, tortuous and opportunistic disease that is AIDS. I will let Drew tell you his own story through his letters that he sent me between January 1984 and December 1994. They constitute a remarkable and valiant testimony of a young man coming to grips with his own destiny and mortality.

The art of correspondence is alive for those of us who still prefer the deliberate stroke of a pen to the keyboard of a computer sending out cursory e-mail messages or using the telephone to talk for hours without often saying too much except exchanging news and bits of conversation. Letters keep. They can be read and re-read over and over again. Letters hold a certain and special intimacy that other forms of communication do not have. They can be held in your hands, touched while the eyes grasp the personal features of the handwriting. They allow for the deliberate process of absorbing for reflection the written word. Letters are the concrete manifestation of an art just about lost nowadays.

The letters that Drew and I exchanged over ten years are not epistles of great literary worth. Rather, they are the growing expression of friendship and respect for the quality of the person that each one embodies. I say growing because you will probably sense with me that Drew's letters grow with time; they grow not only in ways of saying things, but in ways of being the expression of a maturing person. They also "grow" on you as you read them. It may seem strange, but Drew only visited me once during those years and I felt all along that our letters were more sincerely open and more intimate than that face to face meeting. Probably because presence needs to grow also.

I first met Drew as a freshman in the fall semester of 1978 at the newly established University of New England in southern Maine. I was a teacher in the Department of the Humanities. How could one not miss seeing him with his red hair and quasi-impish smile? I don't really remember when I first met Drew to talk to him. I learned that he was majoring in pre-med with the intention of applying to medical school. He had a quiet temperament although he was known to brighten up at parties and on some occasions when a drink or two loosens the tongue and unravels the spirit. He was a bright young man, a courteous and soft-spoken person who did not tolerate violence. He seemed to excel at everything including some sports.

I truly got to know him when he took my "Living French" conversational two-semester course in his senior year. I can honestly say that of all the students I've had in this course in the thirty years I taught, he was an outstanding student whose performance still sticks in my mind. He was highly motivated, loved to learn, came to class prepared and asked questions. His pronunciation, intonation and fluency grew to a level of superiority. Given the chance and resources, I believe that Drew would have mastered the French language and have enjoyed using it in real-life circumstances such as a trip to Paris or Québec City.

He graduated at the top of his class and was chosen as class speaker by his peers for commencement in 1982. Although I had urged him to apply at our own osteopathic medical school, he opted to apply nearer to home making Temple University his ultimate choice. He didn't want to go to an osteopathic school; he never told me why. Unfortunately he was rejected by Temple. That was a severe blow to him. He floundered for a while and began looking around for a career choice always seemingly revolving around the humanities, specifically the fine arts. He knew of my predilection for the Impressionists and that became a common interest that we developed over the years. When he left Maine to return to Pennsylvania, as far as I was concerned, he was just another young graduate who departed leaving fond memories behind with no follow-up or intent of keeping-in-touch correspondence. In the profession of teaching there are those who leave us and we may see them again periodically; others depart never to be heard of again except through the alumni office. I expected little or no correspondence from Drew. At that point, he was an acquaintance, not yet a friend. Unlike the Little Prince and the Fox, we had not "*créé des liens*" [created bonds].

After a failed attempt to maintain a close relationship with a young woman, Drew had, in a way, sealed himself up in his own cocoon waiting for time to heal and change things. I'm the one who initiated the correspondence; I thought he needed some cheering up. I had let two years go by before I finally decided to write to him. I don't know why I waited so long. I suppose I was waiting for him to make the first move. Although I have learned, over the years, to be more aggressive, I still rather wait preferring to respond when someone needs or seeks me. I never like to impose my thoughts, my ideas and feelings on others. I want to give them choices; caring thrives so much better in the free air of choice, in my estimation. That's how genuineness emerges in a true friendship. And, I believe in the serendipitous movement of intuition. When the voice inside moves me, I have learned to listen to it and follow through with its call. That's what I did late 1983. I probably included my first letter in a Christmas card. I don't remember. I wrote to Drew without knowing how he would respond to my letter. He answered and that was the beginning of our correspondence.

I chose not to preface Drew's letters with too many comments and insights from my part preferring to let the reader go through his letters and share the pain and anguish of a young man who learns that the HIV virus may very well kill him. I also chose to include all of his letters to me even those prior to his opening up about his contracting the much-feared and deadly virus, because I wanted to share with the reader the full quality of this young man, my former student, friend and my sharer of dreams, creativity and the fine arts. I also chose not to edit any letter except for a very few spelling corrections and I left his French as is without rewriting it for accuracy; I wanted to preserve authenticity. So, let the epistolary journey begin.

January 3, 1984

Dearest Dr. Beaupré,

Bonjour! J'ai reçu un cadeau incroyable quand j'ai reçu votre lettre [I got an incredible gift when I received your letter]. If I had made any Christmas wishes, they would have included ones to get back in touch with those I had cared so much for in the past but hadn't because I was too embarrassed and too afraid of more rejection. I truly feel blessed that you could be strong enough to do so; I miss your influence immensely and just the glitter of hope that your letter gave me has brightened each day since.

Please excuse both my poor penmanship and my terribly inappropriate French grammar: the penmanship because the first two fingers of my right hand are splinted after my index finger sustained four different fractures while playing hockey; and my French grammar which is rusty from lack of practice and the temporary loss of the influence of my mentor. Both will heal in time!

I'm terribly disappointed that you couldn't reach me while you were in Philadelphia for the convention*. We definitely would have met and gone out and about the town. Did you stay in the Hershey Hotel? It's one of the finest and newest hotels in Philadelphia. I hope everyone was hospitable.

> * *I don't remember what the conference was about, obviously a non-memorable one. One goes to so may conferences in my profession. I did stay at the Hershey Hotel and tried to reach Drew by phone, but there was no answer.*

The coincidence of the timing of your letter and my finally choosing to do some things with my life is seemingly divine! Since graduating, I've really been at a loss for what to do with myself and the longer it dragged on the more compound and complex it became. I lost all direction, motivation and energy-----I felt like nothing and like doing nothing. It was a full-blown identity crisis, like a spider whose legs reached into every aspect of my personality. After spending months looking for help (probably from the wrong people) unsuccessfully, I began to feel like I wasn't worth anyone else's love, concern, influence, help or attention, and abruptly cut myself off from anyone who tried to give me this. Eventually, I bore down and decided that only I could help myself; it wasn't easy but I think I succeeded.

Strangely enough, this is where the break-up.

In any event, what am I doing with myself? Some things have changed, some haven't. I'm not interested in re-applying to Medical School; I still work in the same hospital and the work and my contacts there have driven the desire to continue in the human services right out of me. My three interests are hockey, art, and French language and culture. I'm heavily involved with a local youth hockey organization and have met with more success than I could have predicted. As for the other two interests, most of my productive leisure time has been spent investigating a way to go into a career related to them either combined or separately, and just recently this proved fruitful. I'd like to give Interior Design a trial. To start, every Tuesday in April I'll attend a 3-hour introductory course offered by the local community college. Eventually I'd like to apply to the finest Design schools I can find, either here or abroad. I understand some of the finer schools are in...France! This would be an opportunity to use my creative mind, earn a comfortable living and eventually be self-employed.

For entertainment, I've taken to doing a lot of walking in either the lovely wilderness or in the hectic city, each of which has its own peace and adventure. Also, I've been doing an incredible amount of an old but re-emerging love, writing, a most soothing pastime. But I'm really not as busy as all of this sounds-----I have plenty of idle time but haven't picked up a paintbrush or a French book-----YET!!! I feel like doing it now, however.

Well, I sat down to write a short letter and I now rise having ended this semi-dissertation. Take care of yourself.

Avec amour,
Drew

P.S. I forgot to mention the thing that I'm most jealous of-----your trip to Paris and Nice to study «Les Impressionistes». Can you fit me in your suitcase?*
Bon voyage!

---

* *This was a Winter Term course on French Impressionism that I offered in France to a small group of students. We went to museums and to various sites-----one week in Paris and one week in Nice and its surroundings. We took advantage of the proximity of Renoir's residence at Cagnes-sur-mer to visit this location.*

May 26, 1985

My Dearest Friend,

Greetings! I'm embarrassed to see how long it's been since I've written you, but please don't allow time to mean ignorance----you're in my thoughts and on my mind daily and your spirit has guided me through each day.

I found your last letter very inspirational-----it touched some sensitive nerves, climbed defensive walls and opened closed doors, all that time had buttressed into an insurmountable fortress. I do not hear my voice reading your letter's writing, but your voice expressing our minds's deepest thoughts and evoking its strongest feelings. You are truly an artist----you have opened my mind's eyes, those that have been clouded by misfortune, rejection, anger and other ugly colors of life, and washed them with hope, beauty, love and touch. The past had been something of Mr. Hyde's life, the present of Dr. Jekyll's life. How can I have left my life so devoid of beauty, and how have you so divinely and expertly slapped me in the face to alert me to that?

Much due to your inspiration, I've gone from dragging my feet through each of life's muddy puddles to swimming across some of its widest channels. The decision to seriously approach a career in Interior Design is extremely highly risky. I had to be 100% certain that it is what I wanted because of the financial debts I'll encounter and the time and energy it will take. In order to raise the money to make the initial payment on August

8th, I'm either going to find a second part-time job on evenings and weekends or start working a lot of overtime at my original job. And this is the easy part!

Once school begins on September 30th I'll be working full-time from 11 p.m. to 7 a.m., sleeping for 3 hours, going to school from 12:30 p.m. to 4:30 p.m. 5 days a week, and hopefully sleeping otherwise! Hopefully (again) I can arrange my work 2 days of 5 on the weekend to make it easier to concentrate on school during the week.

Also, by the way, our whole family has moved to a very beautiful township about 10 miles north of Philadelphia...[address]. The offer of hospitality continues to stand if you will be coming to the Philadelphia area.

I've enclosed an article that was in the Philadelphia Inquirer several months ago (on the front page)! I'm surprised at how much attention French language and Culture has been getting lately----but I do enjoy seeing things like this----they make me feel more in touch with the trends.

Now that I've attained my goal of being certain you don't feel forgotten, how has your world been to you? I trust that this time of year continues to be hectic for you, as another year at UNE [*University of New England*] comes to a close. I'm sure the University continues to change and to grow, as you do within and without it. I pray that you are healthy, comfortable and at peace.

For now, be with me in thought and spirit. I think of you and care about you enormously.

    Love,
        Drew

November 12, 1985

Dearest Dr. Beaupré,

Bonjour! Comment allez-vous? I didn't realize how embarrassingly long it has been since I've written you until I re-read your last letter. I must apologize----you most certainly are in my thoughts and your spirit guides me through each day.

Much has changed for me, and I'm not certain where I left off informing you. Excuse my redundancy, if so, but I must fill in some background. My dead-end job at the hospital was getting dangerously intolerable and the plans to go to school for interior design turned out to be financially impossible. Where should I turn next? Frantically, I looked, listened, watched and waited. I went into a local sporting goods store early in June, saw a sign for part-time evening and weekend help wanted, and filled out an application. Four weeks went by, I had given up hope about it, and, to my surprise, was called by the owner (an alumnus of the high school I graduated from), and hired on July 3rd.

For close to three months, I worked two jobs----one I thoroughly enjoyed and one I despised. In September, I approached the owner about working full-time for them and seriously began negotiating financial and technical alternatives. In the midst of this, I was approached by an acquaintance at work and asked if I would like to give a shot at managing their family videotape rental business in a very elite, "well-to-do" section in Philadelphia. Their offer was unbeatable----it still seems like a "once-in-a-lifetime" occurrence----but I was uncertain. Several hours of discussion later, I decided to give it a try.

Since September 30th, I've been managing this thriving business. The hours are long, the responsibilities increased, and the pressures greater. I got off to a slow start but have been accelerating lately. The hardest part of the transition was time; I had been in such a groove from working two jobs that I had a difficult time adjusting to a "shortened" workweek----48 total hours as opposed to 60-70 during the "two-job" era.

Along with the new job, and in the middle of all of this transition, my jalopy died, so I bought a brand-new Chrysler Laser XE, that hopefully will not give me any problems (it hasn't yet!). So, this is the diary of material changes (substantial, I must say) that have caused yet another metamorphosis of my life.

But, the odd hours of free time that I have either early in the morning or late at night have been spent looking through art books, old school books, yearbooks, my artwork, etc. I think it's a very positive sign that I feel happy and fulfilled again when I spend more and more time doing these things. It has been very stimulating and relaxing----and it strikes up fond memories of the past.

How are you? Is there more or less pressure towards the end of the semester?

For now, please be at peace. I'm glad we are together in spirit.

Love,
   Drew

August 7, 1986

Dearest Norman,

Greetings and many congratulations on the granting of your sabbatical*. I don't know if I should offer you my apologies or explanations as to why I haven't kept in touch----but none of them would be a fair or accurate account or rationale. Life continues to be a consecutive series of troubling moments. My outlook on life has not continued to deteriorate however and my attitude always shows that better times are ahead for me. My wish, however, is that when that time comes, all will change. It is very exhausting and degenerating to live a life that is very uncomfortable.

My "new career" is very time consuming. I had boiled it down from a 65-70 hour workweek to a 50-55 hour workweek in May, only to have my 2 assistants quit at the same time. Since then, I've been working 10-11 hours a day, 6 days a week and spending 4-6 hours a day on my day off doing one sort of project or another. I've met many interesting people since our store is in the highest society area of Philadelphia. They all ask the same questions: "How can you do it?" My response is always that "Someday it'll get better." Sometimes my blind hope chokes me.

> * *This was a sabbatical for the fall semester 1986. I spent it in Paris living on rue de Chevreuse in the Montparnasse region. Before leaving, I had offered Drew to join me there for his upcoming vacation.*

Obviously, working so much leaves little time for anything else. I did manage to play on a part-time basis for this past softball season. The other major time consumer is a woman I've now known for 2 years. Our relationship has gotten quite serious and very disturbing. Her name is..., she's going to be 25 at the end of August, she's been divorced and married once and she has a 4 year old daughter. She works at the hospital that I left to go to my current job. To put it bluntly, she's a very common, ordinary, disinteresting and at times demanding woman who was in very desperate need of someone to come along and help with the responsibilities she didn't want and needs she couldn't meet. There I was, a reputable, single and goal-directed young man with enough opening for someone to sink their teeth into. I've been bleeding ever since the bite. I'm not happy with the relationship. I haven't invested much into it, and it is one of those things that will change when everything gets better.

I also have a personal addition to tell you about. He was born on April 28th early in the morning, and he now weighs about 25 pounds. He has blond hair from head to toe (or paws)! He's the Golden Retriever I was given by... for my birthday. I named him "Auggie" after a baseball umpire that was always on the game of the week when I was a youngster; his name was Auggie Donnatelli. He has added much-needed companionship to my life and even more vitality to our new house. We all love him.

And, before I get completely philosophical, I must tell you about a very amazing thing that happened to me in March. I was walking to the bank on South Street, two blocks from our store, which is Philadelphia's equivalent of Greenwich Village. I looked behind me while at the bank and a very familiar face passes by, but I can't get out to approach her. Once finished at the bank, I walk up and down the seven blocks of South Street twice wishing to see this familiar face again. When it looks like another wish will not come true, I'm standing face-to-face with..., 500 miles and 4 years from our UNE experience! We were both flabbergasted. Though we couldn't chat at that moment, we had opportunity to get together when she returned to Philadelphia for a second rotation in her 3rd year medical course. It was very reviving to recount those years, and more so to see that we had both grown in much the same way(that is to say that we had met similar grief and crises). Medical school has not made her a colder and more calculating person; to the contrary, she is a warm, compassionate and tremendously sensitive woman who would be an asset to any profession.

Et, maintenant mon ami, je vous dis des choses que je vivrais(Voulez-vous excuser des fauts gramatique? J'ecris avec beaucoup d'esperes, mais un peu d'intelligence en français!) [And now my friend, I'm telling you things that I would live. Please excuse my grammatical faults. I'm writing in French with a lot of hope, but with only a bit of intelligence]. I've had three overwhelming dreams in my life: to be a doctor, to be a hockey player, and to be alone in a creative ocean with no limits of time, necessity, desire or courage. As you know for now, the first one has been laid to rest. The second is, naturally, laid to rest forever. For the longest time, the third looked impractical, impossible or, outrageous. Now, the desire to do this is so strong it keeps me awake at night and awakens me early each morning. When I first felt it rise, I thought it was just a reaction/defense to run away from all that stresses me. As it grew to the point where I had to pay attention to it, I thought it was boyish.

The motivation for this is a desire for some type of fulfillment in life, a need for adventure, a need to stand out from all the normal run-of-the-mill everyday lives and events, a dream to travel cross country and the necessity for me to return to a creative and stimulating lifestyle. I'm aware of how selfish all this sounds, I'm aware that it will be difficult to convince those close to me that this is real and necessary, but I will explain to all who care what this means to me and why I must do it; if they cannot understand, they must be left behind. I'm aware of the detractors and disbelievers, but they are found in every dream. But most of all, I'm aware of the possibility that I might fail at this, die attempting to achieve it or, that such an achievement will only temporarily change my lifestyle, if it changes it at all. My answers to all of these are simple: if I never make an attempt, I'll have failed disgracefully, if I fail at the attempt, it was not meant to be, if I die making the attempt, I'll have died attempting to make a dream come true (I mean this in a humble, not heroic sense, and if this does not change my lifestyle, that's OK; I live in a style that is a creative desert and a stimulation prison; I have nothing to lose and a lot to gain).

I project that the journey will start in September or October of 1987. I will end when I want it to----if it ever does. I haven't met anyone who understands what I want and why I want it, but I know why----it's personal.

And about your trip to France. I'd love to make my first visit abroad a visit with you. I have one week's vacation coming to me. My parents also offered to pay for a week's visit to Maine as a birthday present to me. I could probably talk them into paying half of the airfare instead. So let's begin planning. I'm shocked that this could be taking place, so please excuse my precociousness!

I'll keep in very close touch with you so we can co-ordinate this. I can't wait. I now have something to look forward to in a more immediate sense.

Thanks for caring. Thanks for thinking of me. Thanks for being a real friend forever.

I love you, mon ami. You're all I have going for me. I thank God that I have you.

Love,
   Drew

October 11, 1986
[mailed to Paris]

Dear Norman,

Greetings! My apologies for the extended "silent treatment"----the motivation to write you seemingly had gone the way of my aborted attempts to come to see you!

Airfare to Paris when I first checked was $758, which would have been fine. While I was awaiting my passport processing, the French government added "VISAs" to the requirements to travel to France*----there is a minimum 4 week wait for those at the moment. I was able to push back my vacation to allow for this, but when I tried to book the flight, the fare had been raised to $1358! Unfortunately, it's too high a price for my one-week dream trip. I (we) have been defeated. I am embarrassed, disgusted and, again, frustrated at the shattering of another opportunity. Can we continue to be «trans-Atlantic» during your stay «en Paris»?

I don't have much eventful to tell you. On Wednesday, October 15th, my one-week vacation begins. I'm not going anywhere (this frustrating statement is not only characteristic of the one week vacation but also telltale of the fear that grows within me daily). Thematically, I've chosen to go in search of the long-lost parts of my character that have withered away from inaction, neglect, unmotivation, cowardness and other assortments of cop-outs. Where have the athlete, the artist, the linguist, the anthropologist and the dreamer gone? Are they asleep forever? If they are, are they dead?

Truthfully, I'm disgusted with what my life is. But disgusted is the wrong word, because that connotes a motivation to change. Hopeless is correct. I'm hopeless about life. There are so many sweeping changes to make that the easiest way to effect them is probably to lay all that I am to rest. Should I start anew or completely give up? I don't believe a thing anyone tells me. I've got no one to talk to (excuse the grammatical error in this statement, please). I'm most successful in breaking longstanding bonds, scaring away opportunities to make new ones, ruining all chances given me. Sarcasm and cynicism color my canvas. Hurt, loneliness, abandonment, distance power the strokes. But the picture is blank when finished. I want to be alone in this state, and the longer this need goes unfulfilled, the more hopeless I get that it ever will.

I wish I could span the distance between us with a brighter ray of light. You are the light of all relationships. Your positive outlook can make anyone happy. Please don't waste it on me.

Peace to you, and to me.

Love,
Drew

* *On a Wednesday afternoon in late September 1986, a half-day off from school for French children, there was a terrorist attack on a popular department store on the rue de Rennes called Tati. A bomb was thrown from a passing car into the main window. Several women and children were seriously hurt. It is after this attack that the French government broadened its visa requirements to include the U.S.A.*

December 19, 1987

Dear Norman,

Merry Christmas and Happy New Year! By coincidence (though I think it was more) I reviewed our correspondence the evening before receiving your card to see if there was anything to touch base on in the "Old Business" category, I got quite a laugh at seeing that the last correspondence you'd received from me was a floral arrangement with no card/name on them ----and you hinted that I could have done this intentionally! That's not so----no matter what my state of mind was at that moment, I would never refuse to acknowledge affections----be they to a man or a woman. They were from me----and that particular florist has lost my business!!!

Your offers to tour with you are becoming more and more difficult to resist. I cannot, however, join you for your sojourn in January, but my spirit and soul will rise beside you in the plane and lie beside you throughout your voyage. This one is particularly appealing because of the subject matter you'll be dealing with----it's very, very close to my soul.* I look forward to recapitulating the trip with you and also to planning to visit you within the coming year----my soul beckons more and more each day to return to Maine to awaken a sleeping portion of my creative soul that is becoming quite, quite restless.

> * *Winter Term 1988 in Paris where I taught a course on French Impressionism.*

I hope your Christmas gift [*a Sensi Write Man kit from Drew*] allows you to continue to write your novel at those times when you're "on a roll," but the materialistic ink gives way. The subject matter reminds me of two French movies I've seen lately that were PHENOMENAL: "Jean de Florette" and "Manon des Sources."** If you haven't seen them, please make it a point----they will definitely inspire some motion in your "WRITING MIND."

I'm also sending you my personal copy of a movie starring Donald Sutherland, Max Von Sydow and a host of other international actors and actresses called "Gauguin: Wolf at the Door." It is singularly the most profound movie I've ever seen about that era, about the seclusion/isolation/suffering that an articulate and creative great encounters and about the creation of a masterpiece from the conception of the idea through the sale of the actual work. I hope it inspires you <u>at least</u> half as much as it did me. There's no hurry to return it, either.

Well, I look forward to hearing from you more often in the future than I've written to you the past. Let's inspire!

Joyeux Noël. Bonne Année. Bon Voyage. Et je t'aime, toujours.

Avec amour,
   Drew+

** *As a matter of fact, I saw both movies in Paris during my sabbatical in 1986 when they first came out. I must have neglected telling Drew about it.*

June 8, 1988

Dearest Norman,

My apologies for such a long interval between writings. Many could be the reasons but none would be acceptable.

How have you been? I trust that you continue your creations, be they in a black/grey/white or technicolor way. The most difficult lesson I've learned in years is the personal greatness and achievements are attainable no matter what the state of my life or mood is at any moment. I've read, heard and been told that some of my favorite French Impressionists/Pointillists painted their greatest masterpieces in times of meagerness, of despair and of ill-health. This serves as inspiration to me just as the brightest idea must come as inspiration to you in a "non-creative" moment.

Please don't take this as meaning that the times of late for me have been characterized my meagerness, despair of ill health----since it's really been quite to the contrary. I have recaptured the ability to see, sense, feel & maintain beauty in life and also have grown it to the point where I can affect the way others can perceive it in their life. If I were to leave this Earth tomorrow, it would be with the peace that you feel knowing you have made a change in others, much like you have done for me. There really isn't a greater gift, a greater accomplishment or a greater compliment I can give you. At some point in my life, I would like to be able to say that I have done as much for you!

Lately, I've lent much thought to what other things I would like to either attempt anew or reproach. The paintbrushes dangle in my mind, the French liaisons* linger in my ears and the time is now. I would not and do not want to look back when I am 80 years old and regret not having spent what will look then like little time to cultivate those God-given and God-forsaken talents. Language and art are the only areas in life that I can "free-spirit"; no essential planning, scheduling, defining or dead-living to deal with unless I choose to.

In late February and early March bordering on and at the verge of "burnout," I took a 10-day sea-kayaking trip to Baja, California, Mexico. The trip's effects are only now proving to be as holistic as ever imaginable. The trip began with an overnight stay in La Paz, Mexico which is at the tip of the Baja, California Peninsula. The following day there was a four-hour bus ride north to Lopez San Mateo, a small fishing village. From there, our group of 12 left on our 8-day journey to watch the migration of the California Gray Whales from kayaks. The trip was grueling, the weather uncooperative but the sights and rewards far outweighed the sweat, FEAR and heartache that took place. At the time of year that we were out there, the females had given birth to their calves and were teaching them the necessary lessons for their 4000-mile journey back to the Alaskan waters. Therefore, we saw, touched, watched and at times played with these incredibly large (40-60 feet) animals.

---

*   *In French phonetics the linking of the final consonants------s or -----x with a mute "h" or a vowel such as, les heures and aux amis.*

They would surface beside the boats to be patted, would playfully "blow" when they surfaced next to us right in our faces, at times would wave their pectoral fins to splash us or flap their flukes to make waves and also "spy"-hopped" right in front of us so we could meet eye-to-eye. Spyhopping is the term given to the whales coming vertically out of the water head first to locate their placement with reference to land. Can you imagine looking up and seeing a 25-foot baby whale standing on its fluke 10 feet in front of you? At one point, we came across a hostile cow who didn't like us getting too close so she proceeded to surface directly under the boat and lift us five feet out of the water.

In any event, none of the people on the trip were known to me. They were from all over the country and we lived and learned together in a truly synergistic way. I didn't do much soul-searching on the trip, but I returned feeling more tranquil, complacent and focused. I've enclosed several pictures* from the trip for you as points of interest. I would have framed the enlargement for you(my favorite shot of the 200 or so that I took) but I wasn't sure of where you might hang it. I think it portrays the tranquility I feel and hope it brings warmth to you each time you look at it.

I've been pondering a trip north between now and the end of October. Would it be possible to see you when I do? Let's discuss it.

Now that I've rambled on for long enough(why is it so difficult to express myself briefly) I'll part for now.

---

* *I received two photos: one a 4 X 6 shot of a whale coming out of the water and the other an enlargement of a desert area with sand and sky.*

Remember this, ———▶ ◀———
Peace to you!

Love,
    Drew

There is a lapse of almost two years when Drew did not write to me. In early 1990, I pleaded with him to communicate with me and the next letter gave me the reason why he had not corresponded with me in such a long time. I must say that 1989 was a very busy year for me what with two trips to Paris: one, a Winter Term course in January, another, a six-week National Endowment for the Humanities Summer grant to study Gothic architecture in l'Ile-de-France. Of course, there were cards exchanged then, but no letters.

April 2, 1990

Cher Norman,

I have read your last letter weekly and the guilt I've overcome by has prompted this writing----as well as any desire to remain in touch with a mentor no matter how far I drift from your influence or how overwhelmed by the many disasters that have besieged my life in the past two years. The first two lines of your last letter read, "I haven't given up on you.....I guess I never will. Just a few words from you would make my day." Norman, expression of any type has become very, very difficult and the act of concentration on the expressions is transcent-at-best.

Since my attention was drawn to the Book of Job in the Holy Bible and to the writing of Victor Hugo's "Les Misérables" while in high school, they have grown in importance from "reading assignments" to living, meaningful sources of hope and guidance for a man who may only live his life on a day-to-day basis and must resort daily to his Quaker/Christian beliefs to maintain this.

Norman, I dedicated my life to my family and to my career and both have failed me. On August 8, 1988, my mother and sister disappeared; they decided to move away from us entirely unexpectedly after 28 years of marriage and completely emptied our house. Two weeks later, my father benignly attempted to commit suicide. Since, he has exacerbated lifelong alcoholism that he refuses treatment for, basing his judgment of the fact that it hasn't interrupted his ability to work or pay bills.

Two of my brothers also live at home with my father and I and, instead of helping to fill the hole created by my mother's and sister's absence, they have only made it wider. I have worked night and day to keep our house, to the point where I am financially insolvent and on the edge of my sanity. In January 1989, I learned that I had been infected by the AIDS virus after helping a man I knew and found in a diabetic coma on the street (a customer of mine at my store) and had been jabbed mistakenly by his syringe once I got him home. He passed away in December 1989 of an AIDS-related disease. At this time, I am asymptomatic but the distress of living with this is paralyzing.

As if this were not enough, after 3-1/2 years of dedicated service to my employer, he closed the business in May, 1989 and reneged on back-pay, severance pay and any help with placement. I have eventually found another job, but the loss of pay and the scarring of 3-1/2 years of wasted dedication continue to burn. And, finally, 2 months before getting engaged to......, my love of 3 years, she has abandoned our relationship.

All of this has created a tremendous loss of my identity. I haven't sought medical consultation for the HIV infection----I pray to God that he bless me with death before all dignity is lost. I am prone to preparing to die and to arranging for my exit from life. I have become introverted, cold, emotionless and impersonal. I am unable to communicate on an interpersonal basis. I am beleaguered by the fact that I'll never have children of my own. I get overwhelmed by the stark reality that, though I am not yet 30, I will soon be preparing a will, making my funeral arrangements and concentrating on these things that I shall leave to my survivors.

I am comforted by warm, glowing memories of relationships past. I live each day as if it will never end and as if there were no reason to live it "normally." I think often of the things I wanted to accomplish with my life and how patient I once was that I had a long life in which to do it. The brevity of the available time now makes me very confused and pressured about what to attempt next, not knowing if there is sufficient time for completion, only to have my concentration destroyed by the fear that no time remains for other things. I have been unable to commit to anything or anyone----I cannot knowingly instill hurt or pain in another human being.

Norman, I must now stop this emotional outpouring, for this is not the purpose of my writing. I have a vacation period around the Independence Day Holiday [during] which I am planning to join a friend of mine who's bicycling across the country as a benefit for the American Lung Association. The trip ends in Boston. I have always wanted to be in Boston for the July 4th festivities. Health and money permitting, I am exploring the idea of meeting him in Boston; I'd like to bike up but will travel otherwise if necessary. I was thinking of continuing on to Maine after the celebration and possibly flying back. I would like to see you----if that's OK, there are some artistic objects----writings, poetry, photography, paintings, etc. which I would like to discuss with you----if that's OK. I don't feel that I know anyone else who might understand what I would like to do with them other than have them destroyed or forgotten, as astutely as you might. If this time of year is not good for you, might you have other suggestions?

I must go now. I am drained and feeling that I am rambling. It is my hope, however, that something I do in my life will, at least in a token sense, show you what I will always carry the torch of your love close to me heart.

Love,
    Drew

May 9, 1990

Cher Ami,

Many thanks for sharing your spiritual prowess with me in a time of tumultuous despair. I'm sure that you're aware that men in my predicament are prone to periods of hopelessness. With the load of other negative circumstances of that moment, my spirits succumbed to the weight.

It is true that I have not been "diagnosed." I have tested positive for the HIV virus, as I had been notified by the American Red Cross after donating my blood in January 1989. I have not sought medical attention since, preferring instead to live a more health-conscious lifestyle in fear of immediate loss of whatever dignity I may have left in life. I do intend to go to medical help, seek spiritual support and make it a priority to become as educated as possible to the holistic approach to conquering this problem. I sense, in my more solitary moments, that the strength of my spirit is growing to the point where I will overcome the fear that the outcome of this interaction will lead to the discovery that I have less time than I ask for in my prayers.

Yes, I do have more goals than those mentioned above. I want to change my living arrangement so that I may live by myself and gain distance from my family and their frustrations. I want to master French language to the point where I can write artistically. I have several paintings conceptualized to put down on a medium. I want to make that bike trip north, to visit you in Maine, to develop our relationship beyond its past qualities and experiences. I have not lost all hope!

I certainly breathed a sigh of relief to hear that the meeting with your new literary/publishing agent left you with a positive feeling. That certainly works to maintain motivational energy which I'm sure wanes at times in lengthy projects such as writing books. I would certainly like to be one of your motivational turbines by spawning creative thought and ideals. Your allusion to some of the sensations of life in Maine emitted numerous waves of nirvana. Do your literary endeavors pique sensations in your own mind? Are colors neon-brightened or light softened? Do scents become pungent or evasive? Is your touch tingling? Can you taste the food, imagine its warmth, wince at its tartness, fear its imminent indigestion? Are the blisters on that hard-working laborer's hands so large and painful that you not only share his pain in your hands, but also share the satisfaction that the end of his hard-day's-work brings.

Write it, mon ami, for our growth into a tree is but a sapling thus far.

Love,
   Drew

June 12, 1990

Cher Norman,

Greetings! How are you? The tone of your last letter gave me a sense that you are/were somewhat fatigued-----I hope that you gain some time to replenish your strength. It's important that you not only work hard but also rest hard. Does Elderhostel still use UNE for summer courses? Are you involved?

Was your trip to Boston to view "Les Misérables" your first opportunity to see that play? I saw the Philadelphia production and found it thoroughly enjoyable.

I am again besieged by another medical problem. On May 26, I was diagnosed with hepatitis-A (non-HIV related) and have been at home since that day. I went through two weeks of jaundice----which has since dissipated----and am now trying to overcome oppressive fatigue that has been leaving me no choice but to sleep 14-16 hours daily. There is no treatment but to rest and let the virus run its course. I have, however, begun supplementing the rest with a high protein diet of fresh fruits and vegetables and vitamin B complex and C. I have felt better in the past two days and have the doctor's clearance to return to work on a part-time basis starting June 18th, for two weeks. It's unclear at this point whether or not I'll be able to follow through with my vacation plans for two reasons----the doctor felt that it wouldn't be medically advisable to do much traveling for fear of causing a relapse, and, though the owner of the business I work for has been very understanding and compassionately continues to pay me while I'm sick, I sense that he will ask me to cancel my vacation plans and work that week. Norman, this is very frustrating to me, to play this waiting game and to leave the control of this decision to things/people other than myself. My dream of seeing you vividly persists. If not as soon as the Independence Day holiday, then another time. This frustration is typical of my life lately; if my prayers are answered, it will not continue forever! I have <u>not</u> lost any hope.

Please stay in touch. I will contact you as soon as I have a more definitive idea of the future.

Je t'aime.

Love, Drew

August 21, 1990

Cher Norman,

Greetings! My pen hasn't run out of ink, there are still mailboxes in New Jersey* and I don't suffer from amnesia----in other words, you're still on my mind! I've been BUSY, BUSY, BUSY. I've been to Rhinelander, Wisconsin and back (by car) in 5 days for my brother's wedding, managed to find my own place to live(to be occupied between now and November), been notified of an opening for me to become a minor league ice hockey referee, and six zillion(not really, but it often seems that many) other things that are all somewhat fulfilling and invigorating but also frustrating in that they haven't allotted much time to maintain the relationships that existed previously.

I hope you're getting some sense of the animation and invigoration with life I'm feeling. When things I perceive are colorful, I think of you, the master teaching the apprentice the fineness of such brush-stroke, this delicacy of each word in a literary sentence and/or the proper style with which one must set the table of life. I find it always perplexing and often amusing also that someone such as yourself can be uninvolved in the everyday drag of my life but still impact the macroscopic perception of it so deeply. It must be LOVE! I know it, you know it, we know it. The suppleness of my chest only covers the vulnerability of my heart and soul.

* *He had moved to Cinnaminson, New Jersey.*

Sometimes, I get inclined to "chase" happiness like the little boy chasing the wayward butterfly----only to find the cocoons of happiness lie at my feet, not in the ever-ethereal atmosphere.

Norman, I've had rough times and I'm sure there are more ahead. We can't fear any rough water and forget the smooth sailing of current seas. When I look back at my life, I want that final breath to be one of contentment and satisfaction, not anger, disdain and despair. I want to experience all things feeling natural to me without denying that they may be a part of me---"this is what I am" as opposed to "this is what I could be."

You truly are the telescope, microscope and the lens through which others may be focused on beauty. Thank GOD for giving you this earthly talent----I do!

Please keep peace and be attentive to any beauty that your eyes may bring you attention towards. It is a characteristic unique to you that I love and that others may love also. Please share it with your world.

Less philosophically, my next letter will be on audiocassette so that you may hear my voice. (Somehow, I find this is like getting to know you again)[*I never got this cassette*]. I hope to be able to make a Northern Trek to Maine(spiritually, I need it) in October. We've had many false alarms but now the time has come! Be persistent if I try to squiggle my way out----remind me that <u>I need it</u>!

'Til next time, take care.

Love,
    Drew

November 3, 1990

Dearest Norman,

Many prolonged and overdue greetings to you. Again, I must "apologize" for such a long "silence" but, as you'll know by the end of this letter, I've been quite busy. I doubt this run-down will capture entirely the extent of craziness of my life since mid-August but it'll give you some clue.

Two weeks prior to Labor Day, a friend of mine told me of another family friend that had a small house in Blackwood NJ that her alcoholic brother once lived in that needed serious repair. Her offer to us was that if we provided the labor, she would provide the materials and let us rent it for $325/month without a security deposit and two months rental abatement. It sounded like a great opportunity. After seeing how badly the house was in disrepair and sensing a new type of challenge, we decided to accept the offer. We worked on it for 4-1/2 weeks at every free minute we had. We decided to gut the building and rebuild from the ground up. Now that we're finished and I can look back on it, I don't think either one of us knew how much work it turned out to be. But it is very comfortable, built to our own ideals, and situated in a somewhat rural area of southern New Jersey, only ½ hour from Philadelphia. We have a huge thoroughbred horse farm behind us that further increases the serenity.

In the midst of working on this house, I traveled to Wisconsin for my brother....'s wedding. My youngest brother......and I drove out and back. The ride was 26 hours each way. We left on Wednesday and drove straight to our destination, traveling along the borders of Lake Superior and Lake Michigan through some of the most expansive areas of the Northwoods. Because some family trouble started while we were there, we left on Saturday afternoon and traveled back across the length of Ontario----what a <u>beautiful</u> province. It has given me the desire to do more long-distance driving----projecting the next trip to Maine between Christmas and New Year's Day.

There are numerous other things occupying my time. I'm over committed in hockey----playing, coaching, league treasurer and now, a fully commissioned referee as well!

Living on my own has been very nice. I have my dog with me and on weekends we've traveled to state parks, beaches and mountains in the area. I've had plenty of opportunity to clear my head of old scars and pains and to plan an agenda for my life. The blocks I felt towards being creative either in writing, painting or otherwise have dwindled to insignificance. I hope that this refereeing develops to a profession. I'm pondering applying to Law School for "Entertainment Law"(based somewhat on recent events with Robert Maplethorpe, recording artists and day-to-day dealings in my current occupation) and I'm setting up Studio space at home to pick the old, dry brushes up and get back to painting.

Norman, you're always an inspiration to me with your compassionate, sensitive perceptions/insights into life. When I talk to God, my first requests are always that he continue to grant you that beauty and that he'll always bestow you with plentiful fruits for your earthly labors and loves.

In peace and love, maintain your faith at all times.

Love,
    Drew

February 14, 1991

Dear Norman,

Greetings! I'm overwhelmed with guilt so I've located an empty notepad and a pen wet with ink and I'll write my "therapeutic" letter to you to attenuate my guilt. How have you been? In checking, I can't believe I've not written since before Christmas but the facts don't lie.

Life has taken on a hectic and breakneck pace which has become more rote than fun, robotic than thoughtful. I've had several circumstances lately that have made me realize how ridiculous and unhealthy this pace is and have begun to furlough a great deal of the excess. As I say, I realize that a defect of my personality may be to over-work myself as I learned from my hepatitis-experience----do not pay any attention to what is good for me.

I have been offered the opportunity to go back to school by the president of our company at the company's expense. He has asked me to apply to the Executive MBA Program at the Wharton School of Business, University of Pennsylvania. It's a dream-like opportunity for me, often tempered by worries that this chance will not come to fruition or that I will succumb to an HIV-illness before completing the 2-year long program. I struggle greatly with what is moral and ethical to do in this situation, but I often finish with the notion that I deserve the chance.

Related to this, I will be forwarding a reference to you for this application under another cover within the next week. I hope that this is not too much of an imposition!

I am scheduled to take the GMAT on Saturday, March 16th. Once the lengthy application is completed, I will do whatever last-minute preparations I can for the [word unclear]. Do you have any suggestions?

Again, guilt has overridden me, since I sense the only reason I write to you is to ask for something. Please allow only me to feel this way.

I look forward to a day when I can spend all its hours on creative binges. It has been quite a while and I fear that "creativity" shall pass away. Few are the chances when both time and energy allow me to do so; many are the thoughts and ideas I could creatively express some day, hopefully before passing away containing them.

Norman, you are like finding a rose among the maelstrom of destruction and on this St. Valentine's Day I wanted to express my spiritual love for you, my friend. All days would be different if we did not share our lives.

In peace, love & happiness,

Sincerely,
Drew

May 19, 1991

Cher Norman,

Comment vas-tu? I hope you are well (and have been well). I assume since it's the end of May that you are busy closing out the end of another academic semester's various chores, assignments, tasks and duties. I certainly hope that, with so many vocational concerns you are able to spend time with the avocational areas that become increasingly important to remain sane in life.

I hope you received the two cards that I sent you----just to let you know that I do think of you and I would soon stop hiding behind that "I'm too busy to write façade."

I'm still planning on returning to school in <u>1992</u>! Because of timing, I was unable to apply to begin the <u>1991</u> program. I did take the GMAT(<u>cold</u>) and ranked in the 75th percentile. Unfortunately, most deadlines for the Executive MBA programs had passed by the time the idea came to fruition. Yes, you will be sent recommendation forms for my applications, if you don't mind.

I am happy to see the arrival of spring. On April 1st, I received a 20% increase in my salary and an offer of a company vehicle. Spring also has meant the end of another hockey season and to my tenure as treasurer of our hockey league. This duty became very time-consuming and tiresome and it is a great relief to be so close to be finished with it. Spring has also allowed me to begin my bicycle ritual on a more routine basis----averaging about

100 miles per week. Physically, this has helped me feel and look better, and since the body and the spirit interrelate, I have also felt much better emotionally.

The next time I write, I will probably have moved again for several reasons. I have had a "falling-out" in my friendship with my roommate and think it is best not to stay. Also, I want to move closer to the region where I am involved so much with hockey, the Bucks County region, northwest of Philadelphia. Hopefully, this should save some wear and tear on me and my car, since I have put 26,000 miles on it in just 9 months!

All else is well with me. I get lonely and/or depressed at times, but I believe these are only two of the pigments that color the picture that is my life.

I have a couple of weeks of vacation to take this summer----my dreams have revealed ongoing chapters of a return trip to New England. Want to help make a small dream come true? I was thinking of a September trip. I'm sure we'll talk more about it as time progresses.

You can write me at the same address if the pen needs to. I'll let you know immediately of a change in my address.

Until then, please keep my love and warmth in the shirt pocket close to your heart.

Love,
    Drew

Christmas Day, 1991

Cher Norman,

Merry Christmas from sunny and warm Fort Lauderdale! I'm midway through a very restive and much-needed vacation. I'm here alone and I drove the 1230 miles myself in 28 hours. The only problem I had on the way down (and it was a recurring one) was the state of Virginia which seems to be under construction from beginning to end. It took me nine hours for that portion of the trip----a total of 300 miles! I'm planning to leave on Monday so I can take my time returning and hopefully miss most of the traffic.

How have you been? Do you have any openings in your French class for the upcoming semester? Are you planning to travel soon?

The past six months (actually nine months) have been an overwhelming travesty. I'm not sure where we left off so I'll briefly recount from the beginning(if there was one). In March, I allowed my company to use my Jeep to transport some things locally. While out, the driver was involved in an accident that damaged the driver's side of the vehicle. I reported the accident to the insurance company and took it back to the dealership to be repaired. It took 10 weeks, a lawsuit, a stolen car report, personal phone calls to the owner of the dealership, threats from the dealership and eight thousand dollars to get it back. Apparently, as the car business is usually wont to do, the dealership subcontracted the work to a body shop who subcontracted to a second body shop who subcontracted to a third(disreputable) body shop and eventually no one could account for a status of the work being done and eventually for the Jeep itself.

While this was going on, I was living in Blackwood, New Jersey with a friend in a small house that we renovated for a family member of a friend of my roommates. That situation was deteriorating also. He stopped paying his portion of the bills, kept bringing some stray cats, and generally made the situation unlivable for me, so I moved.

I got my Jeep back on June 10th and moved back to Philadelphia on June 15th. I looked, over a period of six weeks, at many places and answered numerous advertisements but they were either overpriced, too small, too far removed or disallowed pets (the idea being that I wanted to keep my dog with me). Then I called to answer an ad on a whim at the end of May and it turned out to be perfect. It's a rancher-style house on the very northeastern limit of the city----very close to all of my doings with ice hockey. The man living there is a 33-year old ex-Army veteran. It's his mother's house. The thought that Auggie (my dog) was great, the price was right and so I was set. He works 4 p.m.-12 a.m. so I rarely see him. In any event, I made the move and I've been there since.

Well, in the last week of June the engine of my Jeep died. I had it back for 3 weeks. Thank God I lived in the city now because it would have been impossible to get to work without it. My brother....is a mechanic and told me that it wasn't worth repairing the engine that we should look to buy a used one. It took until the end of <u>October</u> to find one. It isn't generally that difficult to find a used engine but this Jeep was built by AMC in the last year of its existence.

During my Jeep-less period, I had taken to biking the 30-mile round trip to work. It was a beautiful ride that gave me an opportunity to get in shape and also to make some good of this misfortune. On July 12th, a driver blew through a red light and hit me broadside. He did stop afterwards----he had no choice, there were so many witnesses. The damage report: broken heel, L, separated shoulder R, 4 herniated cervical disks, 2 herniated lumbar disks. Rodney Dangerfield coined my motto----"If it weren't for bad luck, I wouldn't have any luck at all." I spent the next 8 weeks with a cast on my left leg, making visits to doctors' offices daily for X-Rays, CT scans, etc. I'm still going to physical therapy three times a week and to my own doctor once a week. The only residual effects of all of this are the frequent stiffness in my left foot which makes it painful to walk and also frequent stiffness and loss of range of motion in my neck. I just recently got medical permission to resume playing and refereeing ice hockey and much to my surprise there has been no effect in that area. Of course, an ambulance chaser(oops, attorney) is involved on my behalf.

While this was taking place, other medical developments took place. My physician isolated complications to the HIV infection, namely chronic acute Hepatitis B and possibly also Hodgkin's disease. I've been to several specialists who all have had the same thing to say----I'll be OK as long as everything is asymptomatic! I've only experienced recurring yeast infection in the genital area, some short-term memory loss and recurrent fever blisters. My blood studies are all within normal limits and the physicians have all said that it is important to stay healthy, eat healthy and live healthy. Some have ventured guestimations into my life expectancy----possibly 10 more years.

So how do I react to the news that living to be 50 is unlikely?, 40 is somewhat possible, that I'll never have children of my own, that I'll never own my own home, that I should see my attorney to have my will written(but I'm only 31 years old, doc) that I should get my life in order, so on and so forth? Well, most of the time I see it as an incredible challenge to defeat. And, to be frank with you, there are times when I find it would be an incredible relief to pass away from this quagmire of earthly misfortunes. I often resort to "Les Misérables" or the Book of Job for consolation and usurping my internal spirit. Please be certain of one thing----I will never force God's hand by taking my own life.

So, Norman, I have rambled and rattled on at length. I will stay in touch and live to write letters of rosier nature and eventually to see you once again.

Joyeux Noël et Bonne Année. Je t'aime toujours,

Avec amour,
    Drew

On September 21, 1992 I found a card from Drew in my campus mailbox. The reading on the card's face exterior reads like this: "It's really hard to have you so far away, and yet we are part of each other because of the things we've experienced and the talks we've shared." The interior of the card reads: "But even though I carry a part of you with me, I long for the time when I'll see you again and we can take up as though we've never been separated at all." Inside the card, Drew wrote, "Bonjour, mon ami. I am in Biddeford, Maine at least until Wednesday. I am staying at the Sleepy Hollow Motel, Room #16! Is there any chance that we can get together before I return? I think the best way of connecting is for you to call the motel and, if I am not in my room, to have a message with the desk about a time that I can meet you in the Decary lobby[at the University]. I look forward to hearing from you.

    Avec amours,
        Drew

This was an unexpected surprise since Drew had not informed me of his imminent arrival. I did call him at the motel and he came to my house where we talked for a while. Then we went out to have an early dinner at a small local restaurant. Our conversation revolved around what I was doing and Drew's trip. I didn't feel comfortable initiating a discussion of his HIV affliction. Besides, he looked healthy and in good spirits. We said our goodbyes, I hugged him and he went back to his motel room. He left for the Bar Harbor/New Brunswick region the next day, at least that was my understanding.

28 September 1992

Cher Norman,

Bonjour, I made it to my final southern destination (Philadelphia) safely. Upon leaving Biddeford, I did in fact head north, then west, not east to Acadia, N.B./Bar Harbor/Mount Desert Isle region but instead to the White Mountains for a trip to the Lost River Gorge, a climb to the pinnacle of the Kingsman Notch and a 65-mile round trip up and down Route 112 through the entire Presidential Range. The climb down into Lost River Gorge and then up the 3/4 mile, 60o grade of Kingsman Notch was exhilarating. I did the Dilly Trail----one of the steepest in the range----I wasn't aware of this until I read the trail map afterwards, but it felt great to conquer it just the same.

It was certainly wonderful to see and visit with ya. In retrospect, I must have been like the ever-questioning toddler in my attitude and I truly hope this didn't give you the opinion that I was disinterested or disapproving of your works, which are appealing to me for their pureness in culture, creativity and imagination. I find it motivating as one who always longs to release the butterflies (*les papillons*?!?) of my creative hemisphere that I have a close and dear friend such as you to look to as an example that it can/does happen and also that by hearing of your other contacts in the artistic world that they too demonstrate that possibility. I feel more on the verge of stepping in that direction now more than ever and I'm sure that you could see that it was partly the reason for my impulsive trip north. Of course, there were other reasons for the trip and obviously one was for very, very introspective reasons.

For a period of time longer than I would like to admit, I've been feeling somewhat dissatisfied with the fruits (and lack of them) that all the time and effort put into my job have yielded. I have been able to concentrate in a mammoth way on improving the business and in fact have been more successful in doing so than I ever would have dreamed possible. But in the drive to "increase the numbers," what was the price? Very high as I'm realizing now. On a material basis, I have a healthy salary ($37K/year), live in a big house, have a wonderful dog (that I couldn't be without his companionship). On a professional basis, I have achieved notoriety, company-wide respect, stature, blah...blah...blah. But when Drew leaves work, what is there? NOTHING! I wanted to start working out more frequently, but held off. I wanted to develop a studio to do more painting, start sculpting, learn wood-carving/burning, but held off. I wanted to spend more time developing friendships and alliances, but didn't have the time. I wanted to take that French conversation course at l'Alliance Française, but didn't have the time. I wanted to spend more time reading at the AIDS library at Philadelphia, but worked or slept on the Saturdays instead. I wanted to join/find an HIV support group, but always found a reason not to.

I felt like the teacher who told her most creative students to sit quietly in a part of the classroom and they obediently did so, then were neglected to the point where they are about to rebel, but have lacked the vehicle to do so. Then the vehicle came along(fear of dying without realizing <u>any</u> of these desires) and the rebellion can no longer be contained. Those most-creative students will not remain still and silent for much longer. I can hear the anthem whispering now, chanting soon and providing the rhythm and beat that will guide me to my next accomplishments in life.

Absurdly, I know that no one passes from this life having achieved all of his dreams. I live for this day however, when these dreams have come true and others are on the horizon. Meeting you in Paris is one, a signed copy of that elusive novel is another, and there will be more. There's a star with your name on it, Norman, and soon its light will shine. There is darkness until it reaches you, and only until it reaches you. Once it does, its rays will shine forever. I know in many ways our love for each other makes my faith in you seem blind and time will show that the blind faith in darkness will yield to the light of your star.

    Love,
        Drew

August 30, 1993

Cher Norman,

Comment allez-vous? My inner sense tells me that you or something is not well so I reach out to you to check. I hope that inner sense is wrong but if it is not, I would like to express my desire to listen.

The ebbs and tides of life's river have been providing me with rapidly changing swift currents, ripples and little still water. I completed a level 3 French Class given by Alliance Française de Philadelphie in May and had planned to continue but have been unable to do that just yet. It was taught by native Frenchmen (women) and for the first 6 of the 10 weeks was incredibly overwhelming and bewildering given to the length of time since I last participated. It was very nice to get back into the culture.

I have been unable to continue for somewhat tragic reasons. I have had two one-week hospital stays in the past ten weeks for a recurrent case of cellulitis in my left leg. The specialist tells me this is not related to the HIV infection but cannot find its cause. The illness is quite nasty----severe headaches, kidney pain, urinary infections, swelling and blueing of the entire leg with less of ability to walk or put any pressure on it, eventually causing clotting and finally a 104-106o fever. The last occurrence began two days into my 11-day vacation. I'm home now and placed on bed rest until September 9th.

Speaking of home, you may notice that I chose to move back to my father's house. He had been out of work since the end of January and was having difficulty making ends meet so I came over to help out. It was a good chance to get out of an undesirable living situation in Philadelphia. I had come home several times to find that my roommate's dog had ransacked my room and chewed up several valuable possessions of mine. He hadn't offered to reimburse me for them or to fix my door to keep his dog out so this, along with some other inadequacies, made me spring at the opportunity. I have been at my father's house since July 1st. I have the two rooms of the second floor----one my bedroom, the other a very comfortable spacious den/studio. I also have all of my gym equipment set up in a separate room in the basement. My dog, Auggie, was able to make the trip with me, though I haven't seen much of him this summer. I rented a house on Long Beach Island, New Jersey with a group of friends for the summer so I've gone there most weekends and sent Auggie to stay with my mother and sister.

Now that I have 8 more days of bed rest, I've been mulling over what paintings and writings to start. I've been keeping a book of ideas, some of them very juicy, but I don't know where to start, I'll probably just close my eyes and chose.

Well, my friend, please write back no matter what the news. I miss you.

Love,
    Drew

I went on sabbatical to London, Berlin then on to Paris from September through December 1993. I don't recall receiving any communications from Drew while away. Then, I received the following long letter.

June 25, 1994 & July 4, 1994
& July 10, 1994

Dear Norman,

    I hope this letter finds you well and let me wish you a "Bonne Anniversaire"[Happy Birthday] before I forget. It's been a while since we've communicated and I'm not sure if that's because I've neglected it being "my turn" or there has been some change in spirit or that you've not been well or whatever. I apologize for any sour feelings and I hope we can overcome them if they exist for I'll need your support on several projects I've begun----more on that later. I've thought about you several times daily and include you in each prayer with the hope that you're alive and well. I have been having a very hard time in life but I didn't want to spend our time portraying the bleakness and dourness of everyday life; now I fear I have lost you too. I guess I have not learned the hard lesson of the "true" artist----creativity exists in all times, periods and moods---good or bad, high or low, bleak or promising, colorful or glib, sullen or energetic. I have been finding reasons <u>not</u> to do important things routinely, maybe as a way of pleading to God to allow me to live longer because my work is not complete.

    Norman, I began writing this letter one week ago on my 34th birthday, first in my journal and then rewriting it to you. I'm using it as an assessment to where I've been, where I'm going and where I am. I think you'll find it interesting.

This is the letter that a young man writes facing his own mortality on possibly his last birthday, a young man once full of vitality and promise, one who lived a family life and a gay life independently, one in denial of the other, a once social and popular fellow, now isolated, even reclusive. This young man is not without a sense of accomplishment for what he has done in his life, nor without gratitude to those who helped, nor without spiritual peace for the time I was given on earth, time in which I made human mistakes that were overcome. I do not regret my life, nor do I live in anger that I could not have more. I would not change it, no earthly being lives forever. I still have goals to accomplish, goals that may seem more mundane in anticipation of my spiritual passing seems to approach because of the deterioration of my physical presence. I have relinquished and acquiesced many things, but not my dignity, though some has been lost in my struggle with AIDS. .....'s [*a college biology teacher*] voice still lives within my guidance----"Adapt, adapt, adapt." As long as I dream and I adapt and I maintain a sense of humor, I live.

I have heard the voices of people known to me both living and deceased, consciously and unconsciously, saying that if anyone could beat this disease, it would be me. The disease cannot be beaten, by me or anyone, until the political, social, ethical, financial-----all----climates are aligned with the only and primary intent of doing so. This is far from the situation presently. I was naïve to believe that all efforts are channeled towards a cure. The cold truth is that AIDS has become an opportunistic business much like the disease is an opportunistic disease. Those who are infected are being exploited by those who are not----pharmaceutical companies selling poorly-tested, side-effect rich, unproven and inadequate but very costly and non-curative treatments and therapies, financial companies looking to swindle those "infected" out of their possessions and those that would be passed on to their loved ones, quack therapists with strategies designed to exhaust your pocketbook before someone empties it, so on and so forth. I also naïvely thought that the quality and sincerity of services to a person with AIDS wasn't more exceptional because of the stigma of the "gay" disease and those in a position to establish and provide these services were non-emphatic, non-approving or unable, or more aggressively felt that "the faggots were getting what they deserved." But I've also seen the ethical reason for it----that the research isn't more well-directed, the services aren't more pointed, etc. because of all the half-ass and inept programs that are already out there <u>taking advantage</u> of a rapidly dying segment of the population. There are people and companies who have stated outright that they choose not to use the afflicted segment as guinea pigs for experimentation and I have grown an immense sense of respect for this view from eye witnessing the foolhardy fallacies of those who are doing it. My belief is that the people, services and companies that have made such an ethical decision are the ones most needed to align the atmospheres and climates on earth for they are able to realize that the quality of life for <u>all</u> on earth prospers from overcoming a plague such as this without prejudice, presumption or pratfall and I've been angered at watching the many modern-day devious and deceptive plots arise for someone to take advantage of my pending/potential death and as you can see it has given me a cynical viewpoint but I now am amused at watching the various guises and costumes present themselves and have been getting pleasure from exposing their foolishness.

Though the tone of the previous passage is cynical, don't interpret this as meaning I've become an overly angry, hostile and bitter person----far from it. One of the physicians of my treatment team gave me some valuable advice about four years ago that I've managed to allow to infiltrate my life on an everyday, every minute way. That advice was to always maintain a positive outlook and to keep my mental presence in tip-top shape for that could overcome many things. So I still pray for a cure (as well as other things), and I still look forward to each day (and those that will follow it!). I'm careful not to be blinded by the reality of the goings on in the world, though.

So, let's now get back to the long, but hopefully interesting diatribe on where I have been, where I am and where I might be going. The sun is setting here on Long Beach Island, New Jersey and the summer horizon slowly changes from gray-blue, to amber to violet. I've spent weekends here for the past two summers with five others and occasionally some of their friends. It's a good chance to spend some time around other people----thank God my housemates (one man, four women) and I are all compatible and within 3 years of age. Though there are occasional conflicts, we overcome whatever comes up and remain good friends. They are aware that I am ill, though not with precisely what affliction; I'm sure they have figured some things out. I would answer and will answer any and all questions truthfully if they ask.

The two summers at the New Jersey shore are a very good indication of all the changes. Last summer was full of activity, sun, fun and partying, but it was tempered by the two occurrences of hospitalization for cellulitis, one in June, the other in August. These were omens that trouble was coming. This summer has been characterized as a summer spent doing very little but relaxing and recuperating from the various medical treatments encountered during the week and what amount I have been able to work at my job, which I miraculously have been able to keep in spite of all you are about to read. (If you've seen the movie "Beaches" with Bette Midler, I have spent the summer much the way her friend did in the movie).

The physical changes began with the second bout of cellulitis. The first bout was unrelated to the HIV infection; the second bout began with cellulitis and then the opportunistic HIV virus had taken over to lead to the onset and rapid progression of disease-related complexes. It began with the mobility to resolve the swelling in my left leg from the second bout of cellulitis there, then the purple spots/lesions, several of which appeared months earlier on other areas of my body, appeared on the inside of the lower half of that leg, just two, each barely the size of a dime. As time went on, the swelling of my left foot increased and began moving up into the ankle and the spots on my leg were growing in size. Other purple lesions began to appear on more-public areas of my body, particularly on the side of my nose which started as a pin-size spot and by November covered the entire left nostril. The purple lesions were diagnosed as Kaposi's Sarcoma, an AIDS-related skin cancer evidenced only in gay and bisexual men afflicted with the HIV-virus----it's the same ARC (AIDS-related complex) exhibited by Tom Hanks in the movie "Philadelphia" if you've seen it.

The treating physicians threw their hands in the air and said there was nothing that could be done to stop the progression of either the swelling in my leg or the purple lesions. The truth of the matter is that there are/were early treatment interventions that could have been done that would have avoided more problems, they just didn't know what they were and wouldn't admit that they didn't know.

I found this very hard to believe so I began my own exploration, half out of insult, and half out of desperation. Aside from the results I've already mentioned, the stark truth was that the physicians of my treatment team, from the primary care physician to the infectious diseases team to the seven other specialists with whom I had been sent on consultation had <u>no</u> training and <u>no</u> education in treating the HIV and didn't seek or send me to consult with anyone who did, all assumed this meant I was progressing to my death and since the disease was incurable, nothing could stop it. Meanwhile, the swelling had increased and elevated up above my knee and the spots on the leg had combined to one and covered the area from my ankle to just below my knee. I couldn't wear shoes without cutting the left one, the girth of my left calf was 7 inches greater than my right one and my left thigh 12 inches greater than my right. It was difficult to fit pants over the leg. In one of the many moments where quackery seemed to infiltrate the realm of medical possibilities, a very prominent vascular surgeon, seeing that the lymph edema (swelling) was progressing rapidly and that the compression stockings were not only <u>not</u> reducing it but were causing it to elevate faster, seriously recommended amputation. Need I say that the pain factor was great enough for me to consider this idea, but not for long. We were able to manage the pain with narcotics which made it easier to live day-to-day.

The one positive result that came from this was advice from one of the doctors during the first hospitalization in June that if the cellulitis did return a second time it would be a life-threatening sign and I should actuate realizing some of the things I wanted to do in life----that a second occurrence significantly reduced the prognosis for life. I was able to play the first half of the hockey season for two teams before it became too much. The exercise actually seemed to flush out the swelling. But eventually the swelling was so great, I couldn't get my skate on. I also became more involved in hockey officiating. This was my fourth season of it and I actually accomplished my A4 rating, meaning that I was a "pro prospect" and received an invitation to go to national select camp in Lake Placid, NY which I politely declined. I also bought a new Jeep(just in time to overcome those four major winter storms) and bought and learned to ride a motorcycle.

The popularity of the movie "Philadelphia" and the ugliness of the KS lesions on my face were making it difficult to "hide" my illness; very few knew the truth and I began feeling compelled to tell the truth to those I chose, like my family, who had not been told the "complete" truth. I made this a priority, but I chose to do it carefully, with the expectation for the worse things to come of it in each situation (which fortunately was overreaction). I also wanted to have support available for my family if they needed or wanted it. My compulsion to disclose the truth grew to adding my employer to the list, since I had been missing a lot of time from work and some "rumors" had started getting back to me that people knew I had AIDS. I chose to be very careful with this disclosure also, wanting to maintain my legal rights. I sought the professional help of a social worker affiliated with the infectious diseases specialists to accomplish these tasks and thus turned out to be the luckiest of connections because he was very helpful with these desires, very well abreast of medical treatment regimes for the various AIDS-related illnesses, very well connected to the physicians who performed them and very motivating to me to carry on with my life and accomplish all I could.

The truth about my situation medically was that it was rare to have developed the Kaposi's Sarcoma secondary to the cellulitis but there were other documented cases that had been treated successfully; several of them here in

Philadelphia by a renowned hematology/oncology team based out of the University of Pennsylvania. The second truth was that KS, though an AIDS-related disease, caused no deaths in and of itself. All documented deaths were due to complications of the onset of tertiary and quaternary opportunistic diseases. The cause of death was either a lack of treatment or failure to tolerate the prescribed, effective treatments(more on this later). These tertiary and quaternary diseases are pneumocystic pneumonia, retinitis and heart, kidney or liver failure. None of these were or are present in my case.

So the game plan for medical treatment became apparent. First, I had to work myself into getting treated by this team from the University of Pennsylvania. That took a lot of work, luck and diplomacy, some of my own money since the health insurance company would not cover the consultation and coordination of calling-in favors and planned diligence and mercenary-like tactics.

Eventually, I had the consultation, the timing of which was pivotal. The swelling had moved completely up my leg and into the abdomen and had been spreading across it to the right leg. The lymph nodes of my left leg were completely blocked and were the size of walnuts. The KS was spreading internally also. Dr......, the hematologist/oncologist from the Univ of PA treatment team told me at the consultation that the analogy to what was happening was similar to a barrel filling itself from within, mine being half-full and that heart, lung, liver and kidney problems usually begin a the 3/4-full mark, which was possibly 1-2 months away if treatment were not begun----but it could definitely be treated successfully. Unfortunately, he mentioned, treatment would have been less radical and more tolerable if it had been started when the progression was obvious several months ago! He did diplomatically mention this in his letter to all of the previous treatment team members at my request. Hopefully, this will benefit someone else in my predicament who crosses their paths in the future.

Our next consultation was about the treatment risks, which were many but unavoidable given the "non-treatment" prognosis. The treatment itself could cause death or one of the tertiary or quaternary diseases with a similar result. I chose to carry on. The treatment was either of two possibilities. First, we would try daily self-injections of alpha-interferon, a naturally occurring immunity hormone with a 30-40% success rate in this situation. However, after 8 weeks of treatment, I was overcome by total exhaustion, the one known side effect. There was also no improvement in the symptoms and the progression continued. I went home and slept almost 20 hours a day for a week; the treatment had been stopped and once this interferon cleared my system, we began the second treatment, conventional combined chemotherapy. This treatment had a higher success rate, a higher risk-rate and a higher short-and long-term side effect rate(the interferon was very low-risk and any side effects were short-term). The chemotherapy treatment also had a higher recurrence rate. The risks were related to the chemotherapy killing the KS cells and healthy cells, including red and white blood cells, which made it increasingly possible for those tertiary and quaternary diseases to occur. It would also cause severe weight loss that might not be able to be stopped, and it could also cause outright heart, lung, kidney or liver failure. There was no way to judge whether I was predisposed to these problems, which concerned me, but I chose to start the chemotherapy.

The two big hurdles were to tolerate the chemotherapy without every organ system failure and abetting the weight loss. The hurdles were high and came in rapid succession. After the third weekly chemotherapy treatment, I had dropped from 195 lbs. to 146 lbs and my GI tract ceased operating from mid-colon down. It was impossible to sleep because of the pressure build-up in my upper GI tract and after 8 days and nights of severe discomfort without relief from anything tried medically, I was admitted into the hospital. This was a known side effect from one of the chemotherapy medications but it was uncommon at my age. After 3 more days of severe pain and failed attempts at causing a bowel movement, the lower GI woke up and things began returning to normal. I was discharged from the hospital after 5 total days looking skeletal at 140 lbs. I was considering that the weight loss was going to continue, that this was the insurmountable hurdle and it was time to lay down and peacefully enter that final sleep.

It's been my plan to enter that slumber when my passing was imminent and with dignity. I had reached a peaceful acceptance that the time had come and was a day or two from acting on it when I had an "out-of-body" experience one evening. I only remember my soul/spirit leaving and re-entering my body----I have no recollection of the trip. I was filled with euphoric resolutions of faith, hope, holism and peace after it. I did not act on my plan.

I have been through 9 chemotherapy treatments, my weight has increased to 165 lbs., there are no free-floating cancer cells in my blood stream, the lesions have lightened or disappeared significantly and the lymph nodes are clean. I have lost most of my hair, 70% of the feeling in my hands and feet (which explains the poor penmanship for which I apologize), I continue to have some severe periodic GI problems that may be a separate issue, and the leg swelling, completely gone 3 weeks ago, has returned but this may be because of failure and scarring of the lymph vessels so we are beginning physical therapy for that. I have overcome, for now! through my explorations into treatments and therapies, I learned about two alternative treatments that I use: acupuncture/traditional Chinese Medicine and herbology. They have both been very helpful.

I also informed all members of my family and maintain, even improved, my relationship with each one. I have also disclosed my illness to my employer. I had expected to be asked to go on disability since I had progressively lost my ability to work full-time but worked in a position that required full-time effort. Surprisingly, my employer decided to change my responsibilities into ones that allow me to work when/as I can with no loss of income or benefits and the advent of a very supportive and understanding presence throughout the company.

And now, I must continue achieving the goals I have set for myself----writing a legal will complete with the proper living wills, powers of attorney and letters of explanation, completion of the design for my patch to be added to the local AIDS quilt after I die, completing the children's books I've started about my dog, Auggie, adaptation of a story I've read for reading at my funeral and/or making into an AIDS presentation public service announcement and some other, smaller projects of personal fulfillment.

How about you? Please write soon.

Love,
    Drew

July 23, 1994

Cher Norman,

    W O W !

You sent a package full of love and energy and I felt it the instant I picked it up at the post office. Thanks. I just kept saying "WOW" while reading your letter over and over. You're on the move, your MS is on the move and your enthusiasm has reached me and probably beyond. Please don't be overly concerned about me----life has changed but it goes on and it goes well. All major humps seem behind me, I've felt good for several straight days and there's much to look forward to----life, not death, is imminent. I'm enjoying the changes----physical, emotional and otherwise. It's almost like a chance to become someone else!

    Also, don't highjack a plane to come to New Jersey. I'll be coming to Maine at the end of Sept. and I hope to visit you as part of the trip. We'll plan more later.

    It's great to hear from you. Write soon (but it need not be weekly!).

    Love,
        Drew

August 17, 1994

Dear Norman,

Bonjour, mon ami, Ça va bien? J'espère que vous êtes bien [How are you? I trust you are well.] I was immediately struck by the beauty of the card you sent last and also by the benefactors of its sale. I think the sale of useful products to consumers is a great way to support worthy causes such as the Alzheimer Association----especially when an Impressionist painting is included! You asked about my own "painting practice" and whether or not it still existed----I'll bring some "pudding" as proof when I head north, then west, in September. I'm planning to spend 2 to 3 weeks traveling at the end of September and beginning of October. I'll be traveling by way of my Jeep and I'm looking forward to the driving. My itinerary for the trip includes stops on Fire Island (on Long Island, New York), Maine to visit you, a nostalgic return to Québec City, a scenic drive through Ontario and finally a visit with my brother and sister-in-law in Wisconsin before heading back east to home. We just learned that my brother and sister-in-law are expecting their second child in May.

Other than this travel plan, the only travel plans were to go back to Florida between Christmas and New Year. Have you any plans to travel abroad? Vous me rendez en France quelque jours? [*I believe he means, Vous m'accompagnerez en France un jour-----I'll be going to France with you some day*] (As an aside, I apologize for any shaky French grammar, diction, etc. Please feel free to correct it when you write back!). ☺

On more serious notes, you inquired about whether chemotherapy was continuing and also about what my plan was for taking care of notifying you and all others of my death. Chemotherapy is continuing though the frequency is decreasing to every two weeks, one treatment of higher doses. On Monday, August 28th, I'm scheduled for the next one and hopefully the <u>last</u> one! ☺ ☺ The opinion is that we've attained maximum benefit, there are no free-floating cancer cells and a CT Scan of my pelvis showed that it was clean. We'll probably plan a monthly or quarterly maintenance chemotherapy to prevent recurrence.

I have written letters to all those when I feel should be notified of my death and the executor of my will is responsible for sending these at that time in a manner that will allow everyone to attend the celebration of my life that I am requesting take place after my death. Of course, Norman, I have written a letter to you too, since you are my mentor, spiritual companion and soulful friend----more of a loved one to me than anyone in the world and one who will never be left out of my life. I hope you know this and my stating it bluntly only serves to reinforce your knowledge. Enough serious talk for now. Another smile has returned to my face as I feel the warmth of the tears being wiped from my face by your spiritual hand as the other rests comfortable and confidently on my shoulder, spreading the aura that this need not be so for a long time. YOU ARE HERE, I feel you!

What have I been doing with myself? I've been reading quite a bit----popular novels such a "Interview With a Vampire" by Anne Rice, medical texts and a birthday gift from my shore-house friends, "Care of the Soul" by Thomas Moore. This last book is very, very deep and I find myself reading <u>each line</u> 2 or 3 times. Need I say that it is some sl-o-o-o-o-w reading but who's in a hurry?

I was also occupied with my brother's wedding on July 15 and entertaining visiting relatives. The wedding was difficult for many reasons and I'm thankful that it's over and I can put all of its bad experiences behind me.

This past weekend I spent at the Woodstock '94 Festival in Saugerties, NY. I survived the foul weather and enjoyed the whole experience immensely. I think it helped reinforce my confidence and ability in spite of all the distractions and disheartening events that occur in Drew.........'s everyday life. Surviving that weekend helps push me in struggles to get up the steps, to take medications even though they don't seem to make me feel any better, to overcome some loss of memory, mental capacity and motor function----just to fight the good fight and pray for a day when there might be even a slight improvement in any of these or other unsavory situations.

I've babbled (is this a real word?) enough for now. Have you any news on your books? It's just a matter of time, Norman, we both know it is.

Love,
 Drew ☺ ☺ ☺

P.S. If you've followed "the bouncing ball," you should have smiled at least 6 times while reading this letter----hopefully more.

Paix,   D.

October 18, 1994

Dearest Norman,

Warmest greetings and salutations. Thank you for continuing to write despite my silence----you should be sure by now that the silence does not mean you are absent from my daily thoughts, meditations and prayers. I also apologize for my inability to carry through on my travel plans as of yet but I promise I'll get up to see you soon. Some unfortunate changes have occurred in my medical status that required putting everything on hold for several weeks and it is once again disruptive to all planning from simple day trip plans and other work plans to weekend and longer travel plans. The condition changes are unfortunate but seemingly haven't altered the positive prognosis on my life. Here's the brief update!

The specialist treating the swelling of my left leg and the oncologist treating the Kaposi's Sarcoma lesions became very concerned with the poorer and poorer response we were getting from their treatment protocols. In fact, the swelling in my left leg was greater than it had ever been measured despite their treatments and the response, which had been excellent over two weeks. They consulted with the HIV/Infectious Disease Specialist and decided to treat what they hypothesized to be another infection in the legs with horse-sized quantities/doses of antibiotics. After 3 weeks of this, the response improved slightly, the swelling receded 10%

and the redness of the upper leg went away. That was something to be happy about! Two mornings later I awoke after a rough, sweaty night's sleep to see about 6 more very small Kaposi's Sarcoma (KS) lesions on my upper left leg, which had been clean previously. That was Thursday. And by the following Monday, when my next chemotherapy was scheduled, they had increased to 200-300. So now we have increased the dosages of the chemotherapy and the frequency from every two weeks to every week also. Added to this is a suspicion now that is has spread to my rectum which has made for some very painful days recently because of the already frequent diarrhea. It's midnight now, I had chemotherapy today and I'm having my usual response to it of being over energized and unable to sleep in spite of taking a sleeping pill and two pain pills. Last week I was awake for 2-1/2 days before I could get to sleep. I hope it doesn't last long this time----sleeplessness tends to begin to produce strange effects on my mental status that make it more difficult to cope.

How am I coping? I cope by keeping my attitude positive, maintaining my sense of humor(a good medicine) and by pushing myself to go to work every day to be productive. In the midst of all of this, I took some time to assess treatments I was undergoing and decided to eliminate some because they were not producing results and were financially cumbersome----my guideline was that if, after 3 months they had not produced the expected improvements or had not helped preventing spread of the KS lesions, they were eliminated. I couldn't continue to waste financial resources, personal strength or trust in wasteful unproven treatments.

Life has been very low key lately and I look forward to the day when it will be less boring and stagnant. My energy level has also been low and life is only work during the day and rest at night and on weekends. Other unfortunate and somewhat bewildering things have happened----my Jeep has been burglarized twice and my stereo and other items stolen from in front of my house. The bank holding my checking account has made some clerical changes to all of their customers' accounts that has caused 15 errors to be made in the last 60 days that have waned my confidence in their competence and this has caused many many problems with those I have written checks to for payment of my bills since the errors have caused complete non-confidence on my part in the bank's accuracy and performance. I think we might have everything corrected by the end of October----after ten weeks of effort.

Good things happen also, however, and I have picked up the watercolors, pastels, acrylics and other media to begin on some concepts. I'm also struggling through your short story* but I'll not write about that until I'm confident that I have a proper understanding of it nor am I asking for your assistance. It's better to struggle and overcome. No spoon-feeding, please.

This past Sunday I made it to the finish line of the 8-mile Philadelphia "From All Walks of Life" AIDS walk. The first half was easy and the second half deadly, but I made it and raised some money in the meantime. We had a team of 35 people from work----of 20,000 or so walkers who raised $925,000 for AIDS education, research & treatment in the Philadelphia/South Jersey. I

---

* *One out of a collection of tales and legends written in French entitled, "Lumineau;" the title of this tale is "Le Cygne de Billie" [Billie's Swan], a magic realism attempt on my part. JCL in Chicoutimi, Québec published "Lumineau" in March 2002*

couldn't keep up with the team but I did finish about 1-1/2 hours behind them with frequent rests.

Well, Norman, my thoughts of seeing and feeling a winter in Maine again are strong. I look forward to progressing towards seeing it true soon----even if just for a weekend. Let's think about it!

Stay well and at peace. Balance your soul and your spirit will fly.

Love,
    Drew

I received the following letter a bit after Christmas as I was preparing to go to Oaxaca, Mexico accompanying a group of students and two other faculty members for a Winter Term course. This was Drew's last letter to me; on the envelope, he had affixed a return address sticker featuring four dogs and one cat put out by the Humane Society of the United States.

December 24, 1994

Cher Norman-----

I apologize for the haste of this quick note but I wanted to drop you a brief line wishing you a Joyeux Noël and Bonne Anniversaire [I believe he meant *Bonne Année*, Happy New Year] before you depart for Mexico. I'll write you at more length later!

I just spent 4 weeks in the hospital in grave condition. I'm home now (since past Tues.) and comfortable. I will convalesce for 2 to 3 weeks then decide what's next for me. Prognosis was not very good at discharge----3 to 6 months----but I feel much better now and feel more improvement each day. Have a fine trip.

    Love,
        Drew

Drew died on Friday, January 27, 1995. He was 34 years and seven months old. His mother called me on the following Sunday afternoon informing me of his death. He died with his mother and other members of the family at his side. With deep pain in her voice, she told me that Drew had died at precisely the same hour as he was born, 7:30 p.m. I was dazed, shocked, speechless. I groped for words that came reluctantly; tears were locked up refusing to come out. I could not stir any emotion; I felt blank. Most of all, I felt cheated, cheated out of a last moment, a last opportunity, a final word with Drew. He had assured me that there was time. I had credulously accepted the notion that minimally three to six months remained and probably even more time. Why hadn't Drew told me about the true severity of the last stage of his illness? Why hadn't he called me to his bedside? After all, I had pleaded with him to allow me that single and precious favor. Why hadn't any member of his family informed me sooner? Why?

It ended up to be a very awkward conversation filled with uncomfortable holes. Afterwards, I felt terrible and somewhat remorseful for not having had a more sympathetic or compassionate response to the mother's call. She briefly informed me of the burial, not mentioning Drew's wish for a celebration of life memorial service. Although she gave me her telephone number, I did not get back to her. Why? I felt as if I had nothing more to tell her and she had nothing more to tell me. I did not attend the funeral. I felt that there was nothing more I could do. Even if I did attend, I would find myself with a group of people who were strangers to me. I could not feel close to people who did not always seem close to Drew. I know they were family to him, but I felt awkward and shy towards them. They had failed Drew so many times. I know that I was partial to Drew and my feelings led me to consider this whole affair with prepossessed feelings, but that's the way I saw things. Drew had let me in on what was happening in his family at various intervals and I did not like the way things worked out for him. He became the victim of so many hurtful circumstances. At times, I called him the bad luck kid. Of course, some of it may have been Drew's fault. I don't know. All I know is that he always seemed to me to be the appeaser, the helpful one, the one who tried to make things work for his entire family and, in the process, suffered much from the lack of true reciprocal love. In the meantime, I waited for that last letter in Drew's will as well as for some artifacts and photos that he had wanted me to look at. Nothing. All I got was silence, and that was my line of action. Frozen silence.

I had sent Drew a small decorated red fabric AIDS heart on a string that I had gotten in Oaxaca. I got two of them as a token gift when I made a contribution to a local AIDS project in Drew's name. Since I did not return home until January 23, I mailed it to him a couple of days later with a letter, my last one to him, that, apparently he never read due to his being in the last stages of a coma.

I don't really know why I saved every card and letter that Drew sent me. I originally did not intend to have them published. I knew in my heart that these letters held some kind of precious and authentic disclosures of a young man afflicted with AIDS. He was living the same pain and anguish that other AIDS victims were living; he was tracing the same steps on this via dolorosa *that other victims were following. Besides, Drew's affliction was not caused by his sexual behavior, if I am to believe his own words. And, I do. Rather, it was triggered by an act of kindness. This really breaks the stereotypic mold of most AIDS victims that we read about. His letters then are the concrete testimony on a contemporary affliction with which, as a world society, we are still struggling with mixed results. In the meantime, people die: men, women, children. And so, I eventually saw in Drew's letters the universal quality of suffering and coming to grips with human destiny and death. My intuition had told me to keep those letters and my presence of mind then told me to do something with them. I'm glad I did.*

In Retrospect

When I think about Drew, I think of a young man who lost his sense of direction and purpose in life. He felt unworthy of the love and concern of others not because he did not need them, but because he felt crushed by life's ironic twists and dead-end happenings. He thus led a life that was "very uncomfortable" and told himself that he wasn't "going anywhere." He often lived with a blind hope and when things did not turn out the way he had planned them, he accepted his fate with discomfort and resignation. He had three dreams, as he stated. The first two were dead and he struggled with the third one only because he could not fit it into his pragmatic way of looking at a career in life. He desperately wanted answers and especially guarantees. He rejected mediocrity, the commonplace and the lack of creativity. He claims that he was living in a "creative desert" and in a "stimulation prison." He reminds me, at times, of a male Madame Bovary. But, most of all, he reminds me of a present-day Job.

Drew makes reference to Job on two occasions: when he first finds out about his being infected with the HIV virus after his family has disintegrated and when he learns about the complications of the infection and knows that he will not live beyond forty. It is interesting also that he resorts to both the Book of Job and Les Misérables. Both protagonists bear the burden of life on their shoulders. Both deal with the onerous sense of injustice. Both are crushed by human fate and can be seen as victims. However, Jean Valjean is a romantic hero while Job is more of a tragic one. While it is true that both enjoy a happy ending, Job wrestles with destiny in a more tragic way. Unlike Jean Valjean, his tragedy is not limited to or tied to his society but extends beyond to a kind of cosmic sphere. Job's case is not the product of a particular time but of all times. It deals with universals at the transcendental level in raising the eternal, everlasting question as to why do good, blameless people suffer.

Drew sought consolation in both works. He saw in them his own image, his own plight: a man hounded by his own destiny and often overwhelmed by it, a term he often uses. However, unlike both literary heroes, Drew did not have time on his side; he never was able to be "full of years," as Job turned out to be. Was Drew a victim? Probably a victim of his own doing, at times. I say that because he often let things and occurrences get in the way of his actions and his dreams. He allowed circumstances and others to crush him. And, I may add, he accepted defeat too easily. True, many things happened to him that were beyond his control, but when an airfare seems prohibitive, there must be ways of finding another more suitable; when the dream of becoming an interior designer is pushed aside because it is "financially impossible," there has to be ways of overcoming any situation if it is costing you your dream. Sometimes I wanted to shake Drew out of his apparent inertia just to make him realize that life need not be that way. He apparently wanted life to be kinder to him. Don't we all? When we are young and filled with promise for a future bright with expectations, then we expect our dreams to come true. Many also feel that if one is true to life's expectations of honesty, dutifulness, integrity, and all other virtues demanded of us, then the just rewards in life will ensue. But the age-old question persists, is there justice in this world? This is precisely the question I hear Drew asking at times. Justice is for platonic idealists. And Drew was certainly an idealist. Should we fault him for that? What would the world be without idealism? Without dreams? What would life be if it were only filled with substantiality? Worse, mediocrity, a question that I usually raise with my students when reading <u>Madame Bovary</u>.

I understood Drew so very well, his dreams, his idealism, his love of beauty. This is also my domain. Furthermore, I feel for him when life's journey turns out to be tumultuous, bumpy, scary and so often dead-ended. I never heard him complain or whine; he picked himself up and started over again. As I read and re-read his letters, I felt all along that in spite of his own awareness of failure and hopelessness, Drew never lost his sense of wonderment. He was able to overcome his fear and despair by recovering his capacity to be aroused by the awe-inspiring be it a painting, the beauty of Ontario, the conquering of the Dilly Trail in the Lost River Gorge, or watching the migration of the California Gray Whales from a kayak. All of this helped to fill the emptiness within.

Moreover, success was very important to him, so were relationships. Both seemed to slip away from his hands. Notwithstanding all of his troubles and bad luck, Drew could always manage to find a way out and look forward to a new day. However, the severest and most cruel blow was when he learned he was infected with the HIV virus. That can devastate any man. When youth cries out to be heard and wants its turn at success and the realization of dreams, then the snuffing out of the potential of both is definitely a cruel blow. We who are not afflicted with this deadly plague can try to think about its debilitating effects and its sorrowful message of pending death, but we do not really know what it's all about. We are not the ones with the pain of knowing that we are soon to die. Like being on a sinking ship. Helpless. We are not living the terrible nightmare.

What I admire most about Drew's keen sense of observation and self-scrutiny is the way he deals with his debilitating illness. His clinical account of and perceptions on the various stages of his infection as well as his observations and comments on the way the system failed him and others afflicted with HIV/AIDS are enlightening and strikingly objective. His clear sense of evaluating the system, as he calls it, uncovers the dilemma of a society's stated purpose of clinical awareness and intent of pursuing a cure with its lack of commitment and an inadequacy of ethical perspectives on priorities vis-à-vis the AIDS victim's right to expect competent medical care. When Drew writes, "This disease cannot be beaten, by me or anyone, until the political, social, ethical, financial--------all-------climates are aligned with the only and primary intent in doing so," I fully agree with him. In the meantime, eleven years have elapsed since Drew's death and things haven't really changed much.

As to his having AIDS and the way he contracted it may certainly be, for some, a bone of contention. What was really Drew's lifestyle? some may ask. Gay, bisexual or straight? In one of his letters, he speaks of "living a family life and a gay life independently." As naïve as I was then, I took this to mean a happy life. I never asked him if he was gay; it didn't matter to me. Gay or straight, Drew was Drew and I loved the person that he was. We had so many things in common: the love of the French language, Impressionist painting, books, nature, love of animals, esthetics, and creativity. These things were sufficient in themselves to bond us together and make our friendship a close one in spite of the many miles that separated us and the spottiness and even infrequency of our correspondence. The letters went and came. He knew that I was there and I never faltered in keeping him close to my thoughts. I truly and sincerely cared for Drew and I believe he knew that. I didn't want to invade his private life. I felt that whatever the situation, whatever the circumstances, and whatever the problem, if it was important enough, he would open up to me on all counts. Of course, he might have been reluctant to do so since there are things we keep to ourselves. I was, after all, his former teacher and he considered me to be his mentor. He respected me and held me in esteem. I realize that. So, he might have been uncomfortable in broaching the subject of sexual orientation with me. And I wasn't sharp enough nor cognizant enough of his day-to-day living to discuss his veiled messages if there were some. Today, after I read and reread several times his letters, I'm almost convinced that Drew struggled with gay feelings and may have acted on them at some time. That, I don't know. Be it as it may, sexual orientation never preoccupied my mind when it came to Drew. It did not really matter. I preferred trying to console him and encourage him, and above all, to nurture the gift of inspiration and creativity in him. Moreover, I appealed to his deep sense of spirituality so that he might ultimately find some sense of justice and meaningfulness he was so earnestly looking for. Spirituality, this leap of transcendence, can provide some measure of hope in our lives, since it is part of a holistic approach to healing. The spirit can truly soar above and beyond one's sense of vulnerability to illness. It somehow casts glimmers of soothing light on our inner selves just like the splendid hues of colors in a stained glass window radiant with the sun that captures one's sense of awe. I know. I never fail to go to Notre-Dame cathedral when I'm in Paris, on a bright sunny day, and just sit there to watch serenely the huge rose window to the right of the main altar. I seem to waft on the brilliance of colors so marvelously designed by the medieval artist-glazier. The delicate purplish color, this mauve, has such a healing effect on me. It heals because it produces an uplifting that is both esthetic and spiritual.

I remember writing him long, very long letters, ten, fifteen pages and sharing with him my adventures, my dreams and my work while encouraging him to find his own adventures and dreaming his own dreams. I tried to encourage him in his low moments and rejoice with him in the high ones. Correspondence provided me the ease with which I could weave my thought into words. I have always loved words, the nuances of words, and especially the transformative essence of metaphors. Through the process of time that ten years of correspondence represents, I came to realize that my letters mattered to Drew. They seemed to pull him out of the doldrums that penetrated his life. That alone was worth my writing to him.

What I feel most frustrated about is the fact that time was not on his side, it was not on our side as friends and correspondents. Time is a slippery evader. It often fills us with the illusion that it will be generous and will give of itself to us especially when it is painfully needed. I was wrong. I was even naively under the illusion that I had enough time to deal with Drew's departure from life. He knew he was dying and I knew it; we did not have any illusion about death in this case. But, basing myself on Drew's words and feelings, I felt that if he wanted me there he would call for me. I also turned down many an opportunity to either write to him or call him. I should have gone to his motel room that night when he visited me in 1992. I should not have been satisfied with a few hours of civil and friendly talk. I should have gone there to really talk to him. But of course, I figured there would always be time, later on.

Why did I feel cheated when I heard of his death? After all, I should have seen it coming when he wrote me his last letter. I felt cheated because I had cheated myself by thinking that time was a luxury. I felt angry at myself for not doing enough when the opportunities presented themselves. How many things and how many lives would be altered if only we could, in retrospect, change things. But we cannot. That's the infuriating and frustrating thing about life. We make it that way, and we don't seem to learn. The one thing that I have learned from this are those age old words, *carpe diem*. Do it now, don't wait for time. Go beyond intentions; go directly to action. Rationalization and procrastination are two of the stultifying aspects of human nature that congeal the flow of our determination to act. I need to listen more and more to my soul, my intuition and my inner voice.

For months and even years, I relegated my writing about Drew in the back of my mind since the manuscript was not yet complete, so I thought. I felt I needed to talk to Drew's mother about her son's end of life. I needed to add more details so that the reader would not have to ask whether the story was complete or not. Why didn't I follow up on it was my imaginary question from the reader's perspective Well, I would have had to call the mother and ask her about the last stages of Drew's life. That would certainly have reopened some painful wounds. Besides, as time went by, I tended to feel more and more awkward about reaching her. Perhaps, I told myself, it was too painful for both her and me. It was perhaps better left unsaid. What more would it add to the meaningful reality of my writing about my dear young friend? More details about Drew"s death? What for? Also, ask the mother whether her son was gay or not? What for? I also wanted sincerely to protect Drew's family's privacy since he had revealed to me some serious family wounds. I decided to leave Drew and his death wrapped in his own sense of dignity and quiet reverence.

As for AIDS, I have now lost two very good friends to it. One was a poet and a teacher who died in his early fifties and Drew. It's not a gay disease. It's a people affliction. It's not just the poor people in Africa and Haiti. It's here. Over all, few survive and so many are taken away from us in the very prime of their lives. We tend to think that it's not fair. What is fair? Death is not a chastisement, nor a penalty for a life not led according to some fundamental principles, nor is it the end of all being. As Native-Americans have long looked at it, death is but a normal and natural part of life. But we human beings that we are see suffering and pain, death and end-of-life experiences, especially for young people, as torment or injustice. I truly believe that Drew healed himself and was reconciled with death. He healed because he was able to gather all of the incongruent parts within himself and ultimately effect a deep harmony. The out-of-body experience that he says he had manifests this harmony to me. With time, I got to heal too. My healing came with his healing. Somehow, I was able to reconcile death, life and suffering as one full circle [like the shamanic *uroborous*; shamanic healing]. In Christian terms, the full circle of redeeming love. I no longer seek understanding, but inner harmony. I miss him, I miss our written conversations about creativity, aesthetics, dreams, travels and the intellectual and imaginative challenge of the mind. I still feel his presence within me. His soul is at peace now, a quality of being he always sought. Full, holistic, penetrating peace seems to be the answer to the Job question of the why. As for the why in my case, why didn't Drew call for me before the very end, my answer comes from the deep feeling inside me that he did not want me to see him that way, emaciated, haggard and drained of all life. But a shadow of the Drew I once knew. He did not want me to gasp at his full and open vulnerability close to death. At the very least, he wanted to maintain and cling to a part of his dignity. And, I understand. I miss him deeply but I no longer grieve him. He has found his serenity, his soul-love and his beatitude. I look for you in the stars, my dear friend.

LaVergne, TN USA
19 August 2009
155286LV00001B/70/A